T0381148

INVISIBLE

NEUSA CORREIA LOPES

To order additional copies of this book, contact:
Xlibris
844-714-8691
www.Xlibris.com
Orders@Xlibris.com

ISBN: Softcover   978-1-6698-3773-2
        EBook   978-1-6698-3774-9

Print information available on the last page

Rev. date: 07/19/2022

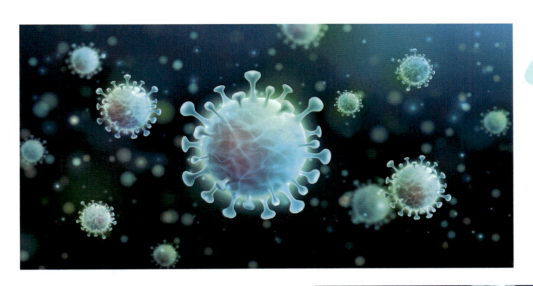
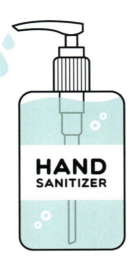
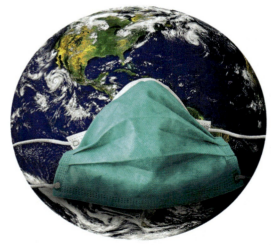
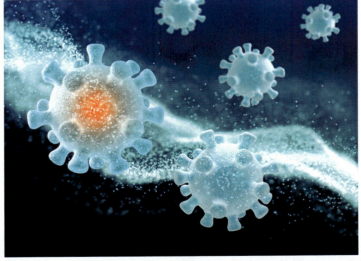

Invisible

Is a biannual magazine that brings you updates about education and its accommodation, challenges, and changes throughout this PANDEMIC. This magazine will bring you to reflect on the changes and the challenges that we educators, teachers, professors, parents, and students are going through. This magazine will also put the readers to reflect on its updated puzzle.

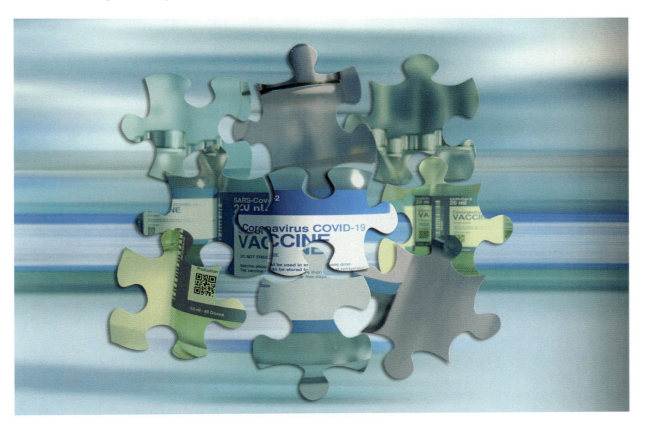

We Have Learned...

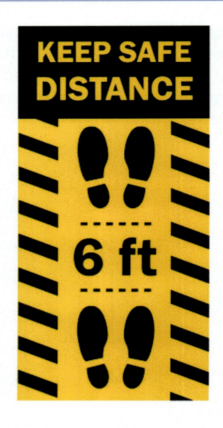

Stay six feet away while in school!

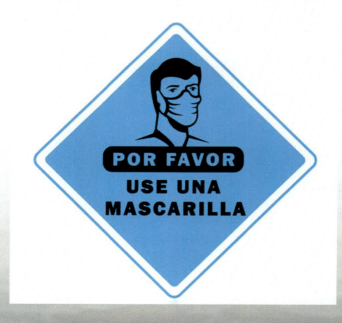

Signs about wearing masks are in all languages.

Coronavirus

This virus has been portraying the world and the Education Realm by puzzling with its variant in the classroom setting.

What are they?

"Coronaviruses (CoV) are a large family of viruses that cause illnesses ranging from the common cold to more severe diseases. A novel Coronavirus (nCoV) is a new strain that has not been previously identified in humans."

http://www.euro.who.int /en/healthtopics/health-emergencies/coronavirus-COVID.

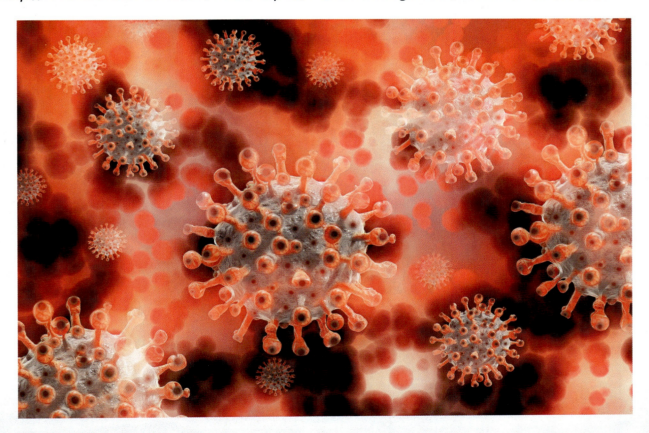

Covid-19

"Illness caused by SARS-CoV-2 was termed COVID-19 by the WHO, the acronym derived from "coronavirus disease 2019." The name was chosen to avoid stigmatizing the virus's origins in terms of populations, geography, or animal associations". http://www.euro.who. int /en/healthtopics/health-emergencies/coronavirus-COVID.

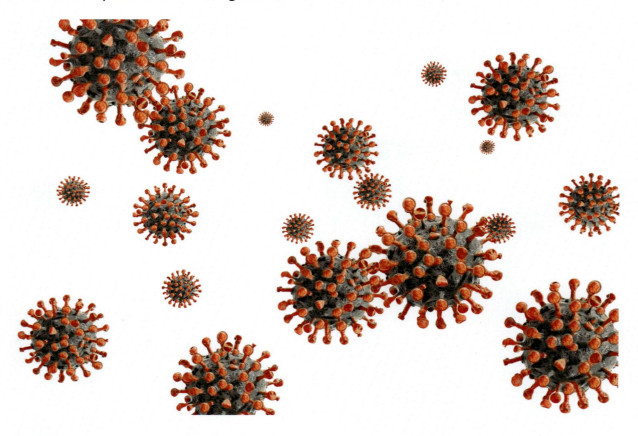

Surfaces Contacts Vs Coronavirus Disease

According to scientists: "Our skin has hydrophobic properties similar to those of the lipid. The membrane of the virus consequently, the coronavirus sticks to our skin better than surfaces in your home, so that when we touch a contaminated surface the virus lifts off and sticks to our hands instead. Warm water does not contain surfactants and, when used alone, it is less effective at lifting the virus off household surfaces or our hands compared to washing hands with soapy water"

READERS REFLECTION

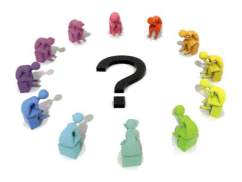

How can we educators protect ourselves from Coronavirus in the education realm?

_____

_____

_____

_____

_____

_____

_____

_____

Scientists have proven that: "the most effective method of controlling the spread of the virus is through good hygiene and decontamination practices does disinfect surfaces for Corona virus work for disease control and prevention?"

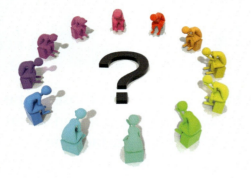

What is your comment on this statement?

_____

_____

_____

_____

_____

_____

_____

_____

We are all living in a society where everyone is worried about the Coronavirus and its variant.

This leads us to be aware of our surroundings. Coronavirus has played an important role in Human Being in terms of being aware of our own lifestyles.

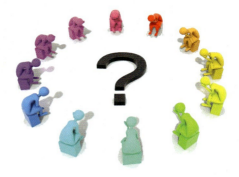

Should we continue to watch out for our diet?

_____

_____

_____

_____

_____

_____

_____

_____

Zoom Classroom

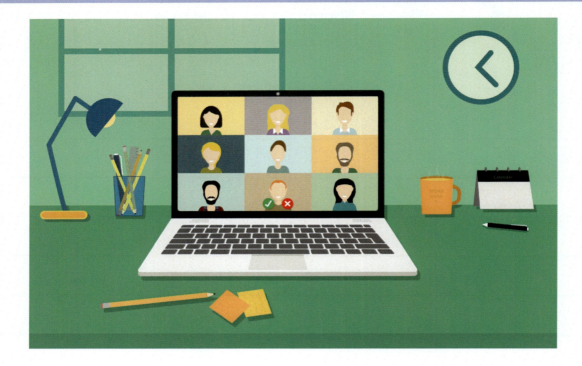

While having distance learning through zoom classroom there will be no problem it is learning of course.

On the other hand, other difficulties in showing materials when ADAPTATION, are needed. Adaptation on how to project the lesson for students to gain the information with less frustration. It is all a big process that includes emotional, social, and psychological as well. Emotional because it is all about preparing ourselves for the unknown dimension. It becomes social because there is no social versus physical contact, this becomes a virtual social life. Where students can go to breakout rooms for group chats or virtual group work. In the end, we have the frustration when students misunderstand the lesson or say: "teacher I can get it. The teacher has to adapt a virtual strategy that can better serve the student to input information to deescalate students' anxiety or frustration. According to Harvard College, it highlights that: *"The Undergraduate Council's Student Experience Survey examined student's experience with the transition from classroom to online learning in the Spring of 2020 secondary to the Covid-19 pandemic. Among other findings, undergraduates Jenny Gan and Oliver York found that "students reported that their overall emotional and physical health has declined. Nearly half of those surveyed reported that their physical health has worsened, and 81.1 percent of those surveyed reporting their emotional health has worsened."*(Sharon xu, Crimson staff writer, Harvard students Report Strain of Online Semester in Undergrad Council Survey,) 2020.

In *"Relationship between Students' Emotional Intelligence, Social Bond, and Interactions in Online Learning"*, Han and Johnson conducted a study to understand how emotional intelligence and behavior, such as the understanding of facial expressions, affect the social bond between peers and their behaviors in online classroom environments (Han& Johnson, 2012). They found a positive correlation between students' emotional intelligence and their social bonds with peers in virtual environments (Han & Johnson, 2012)".

I wear the mask to teach, to input information to students. I have noticed that it is difficult to demonstrate facial expressions especially when the students are foreigners. There is a need for students to see your facial expressions. Teaching and learning appear to have a gap between social and emotional behavior.

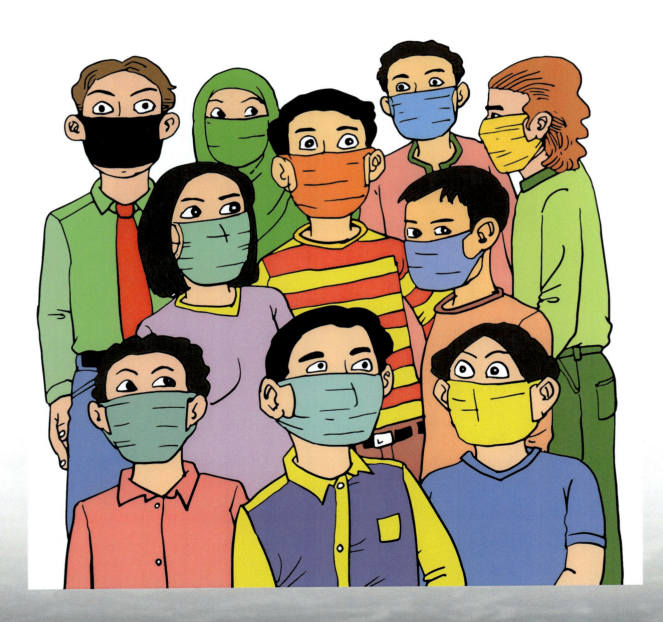

Puzzling the changes, from the virtual zoom classroom to the face-to-face classroom where the digital becomes a crucial tool.

A smartboard helps us teachers accommodate and incorporate our daily lesson plan in an adaptable way to the teaching and learning environment. Its manageable skills such as ESL virtual games, quizzes, and more.

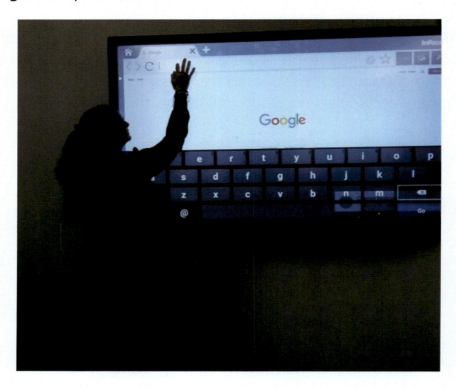

The Use of Mask

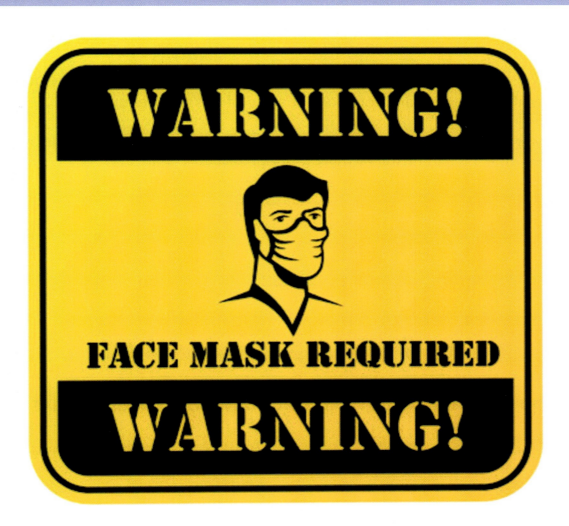

Mask turns out to be a crucial public tool. No matter if one is vaccinated or not, this tool becomes one of the most important for society. According to CDC: "Masks offer protection against all variants. CDC continues to recommend wearing a mask in public indoor settings in areas of substantial or high, community transmission, regardless of vaccination status.

CDC provides advice about masks for people who want to learn more about what is right for them depending on their circumstances".

In fact, the use of masks is crucial and mandated, and it reduces the risk of infection. In addition, it has been the WHO recommendation for the world since the beginning of the pandemic as we go through the pandemic period time.

Students and school staff are mandated to use masks in schools and outdoors during school.Just as CDC acknowledges: "Masks offer protection against all variants. CDC continues to recommend wearing a mask in public indoor settings in areas of substantial or high community transmission, regardless of vaccination status. CDC provides advice about masks for people who want to learn more about what type of mask is right for them depending on their circumstances"

Mask brings us to reflect that society is in danger if one does not obey the government mandates. Many people are not taking the use of this tool seriously.

This may and can be dangerous for everyone. As we all know by now, it is by covering our mouth that we can protect others and ourselves.

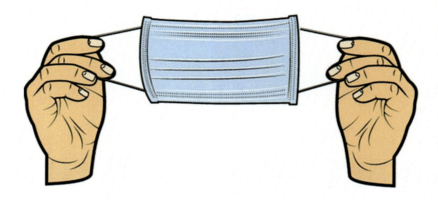

WHAT DO YOU THINK ABOUT THE IMPORTANCE OF WEARING A MASK?

_____

_____

_____

_____

_____

_____

_____

_____

Once again, this mask brings us to reflect that societies are in danger if one does not obey the government mandates. As a matter of fact, as researchers encounter: "many people are not taking the use of this tool seriously". Going back to face-to-face class now, students tend to uncover their faces because of the free masks in some places.

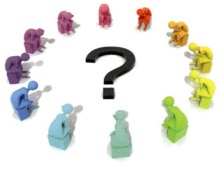 **What is your opinion on that?**

_____

_____

_____

_____

_____

_____

_____

_____

ACCOMMODATION, ACCOMMODATION, ACCOMMODATION.

This is what teachers, professors, and educators are doing. Some students are complaining about it.

This is what I found out when I did my recent research on some of my students when I interviewed them by raising questions about how do they feel during the classroom period under the mask?

- " I can't breathe"

- "I am asthmatic and I feel like I want to breath"

- "Sometimes I feel pain behind my ears because of the mask."

- "I feel okay because now I feel used to the mask"

- "I want to breathe normally".

All of these answers can put us reflect on what can we expect from our emotional states.

As a human being. There is a need for breathing. There is a need for students to see their teachers 'Facial expressions when teaching language is taught especially ESOL/ESL, EFL Etc. Well, there is a need for students while teaching pronunciation, to see how the teacher expresses herself/himself.

Masks are respected for each others' safety. Face-to-face teaching and learning must respect the Corona Virus and its variants.

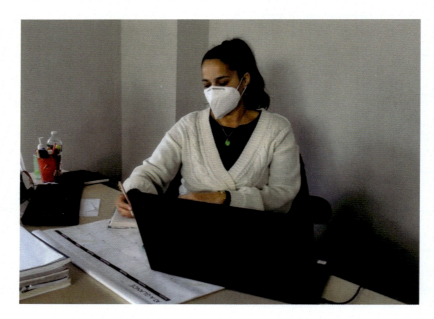

The use of masks become crucial indoors in crowded places. It is to highlight that the use of the mask must and should be used correctly to protect others and ourselves as well. Researchers point out: **"Consistent and Correct *Mask Use when* *teachers, staff, and students consistently and correctly wear a mask, they protect others as well as themselves. Especially important indoors and in crowded settings, when physical distancing cannot be maintained"*.

- ***"Indoors****: CDC recommends indoor masking for all* individuals ages 2 years and older, including students, teachers, staff, and visitors, regardless of vaccination status"*.

- *"**Outdoors**: In general, people do not need to wear masks when outdoors.*

  CDC recommends that people who are not fully vaccinated wear a mask in crowded outdoor settings or during activities that involve sustained close contact with other people. Fully vaccinated people might choose to wear a mask in crowded outdoor settings, especially if they or someone in their household is immune-compromised".

  "*Exceptions can be made for the following categories of people:

- *A person who cannot wear a mask, or cannot safely wear a mask, because of a disability as defined by the Americans with Disabilities Act (ADA) (42 U.S.C. 12101 et seq.). Discuss the possibility of reasonable accommodation of external icons with workers who are unable to wear or have difficulty wearing certain types of masks because of a disability".*

MASKS AND PUBLIC TRANSPORTATION VS SCHOOL BUS.

As I ride public transportation, I can see now that everyone is protecting themselves by covering their faces (nose and mouth) inside the buses, and trains. I observe the worries on people's faces as the mask becomes an important tool in their lives. People also complaint about any individual on the bus or train without wearing a mask. Indeed, being without a mask became a threat to the other individual. According to CDC: *"During school transportation: CDC The order applies to all public transportation conveyances including school buses. Passengers and drivers must wear a mask on school buses, including on buses operated by public and private school systems, regardless of vaccination status, subject to the exclusions and exemptions in CDC's Order. Schools should provide masks to those students who need them (including on buses), such as for students who forgot to bring their masks or whose families are unable to afford them. No disciplinary action should be taken against a student who does not have a mask, as described in the U.S. Department of Education COVID-19 Handbook, Volume."https:// www.cdc.gov/coronavirus/2019-ncov/community/schools-childcare/k-12-guidance. html#mask-use*

Social Distance

Having the lockdown ended and with the openings of schools and public places, purposely, physical distance should be considered one the most important behavioral matter. Social distance should have attention.

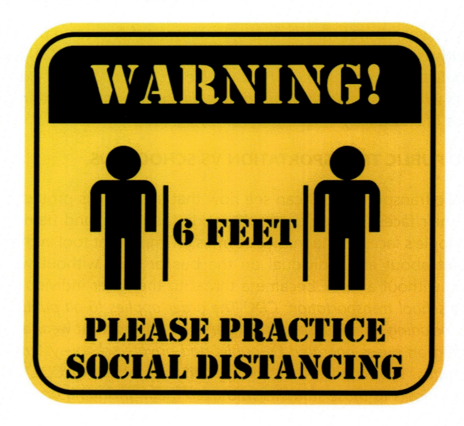

social distance is a way that students, teachers, and staff must maintain during school periods and after school hours.

People have to be giving some space to each other. The distance space becomes crucial between people in terms of people having contact with each other, no more shaking hands. The way of saying hello to each other has changed.

Signs of social distancing are everywhere. The signs of social distance are everywhere, not everybody is respecting it. Some people forget and step over it and go on. Human beings are not trained to adapt so rapidly to a situation that is completely unknown to us. Sometimes adaptation and accommodation are needed. "Social-emotional learning (SEL), defined by The National Conference of State Legislators, "refers to a wide range of skills, attitudes, and behaviors that can affect a student's success in school and life.

Critical thinking, managing emotions, working through conflicts, decision making, and teamwork are all skills not necessarily measured by tests, though they are crucial components of a student's education. These skills may impact his/her academic success, employability, self-esteem, relationships, as well as civic and community engagement" ("Social and Emotional Learning,"2018). In schools, students sometimes forget to do social distancing. In fact, the more the students make a social distance the more they are distant from their emotional capacity of feeling the human heart. Consequently, this may cause some frustration in terms of trying to adapt to the new behavior of Social Distance signs in schools.

Physical Distancing

Experts think that: "Because of the importance of in-person learning, schools should implement physical distancing to the extent possible within their structures but should not exclude students from in-person learning to keep a minimum distance requirement. In general, CDC recommends people who are not fully vaccinated maintain a physical distance of at least 6 feet from other people who are not in their household. However, several studies on the 2020-2021 school year show low COVID-19 transmission levels among students in schools that had less then 6 feet of physical distance when the school implemented and layered other prevention strategies, such as the use of masks."

"Based on studies from the 2020-2021 school year, CDC recommends schools maintain at least 3 feet of physical distance between students within classrooms, combined with indoor mask-wearing to reduce transmission risk. When it is not possible to maintain a physical distance of at least 3 feet, such as when schools cannot fully re-open while maintaining these distances, it is especially important to layer multiple other prevention strategies, such as screening testing, cohort, improved ventilation, handwashing and covering coughs and sneezes, staying home when sick with symptoms of infectious illness including COVID-19, and regular cleaning to help reduce transmission risk."

"A distance of at least 6 feet is recommended between students and teachers/staff, and between teachers/staff who are not fully vaccinated. Correct and consistent mask use by all* students, teachers, staff, and visitors is particularly important when physical distance cannot be maintained.

Cohorting: means keeping people together in a small group and having each group stay together throughout an entire day. Cohorts can be used to limit the number of students, teachers, and staff who come in contact with each other, especially when it is challenging to maintain physical distancing, such as among young children, and particularly in areas of moderate-to-high transmission levels."

Cohorts are done in an equitable way so that students can feel that they are not being discriminated. It is crucial to take that into consideration when the school decides to do a cohorts group. As a matter of fact, we have to respect what is written in the U.S. Department of Education COVID-19 Handbook, Volume1

"The use of cohorts can limit the spread of COVID-19 between cohorts but should not replace other prevention measures within each group. Cohorts people who are fully vaccinated and people who are not fully vaccinated into separate cohorts is not recommended. It is a school's responsibility to ensure that cohorts are done in an equitable manner that does not perpetuate academic, racial, or other racking, as described in the U.S. Department of Education COVID-19 Handbook, Volume 1 ."

Adaptation and accommodation thought us how to begin a new normal in the school environment.

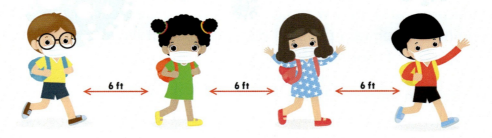

Social distancing.

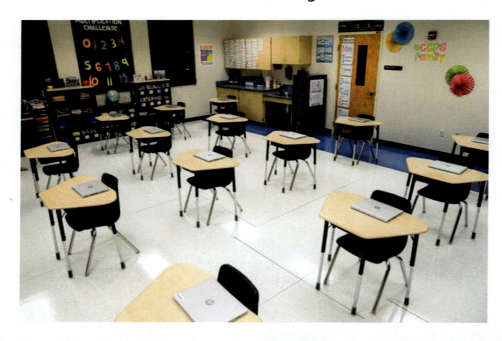

Chrome books are in use at all desks.

Individualism....

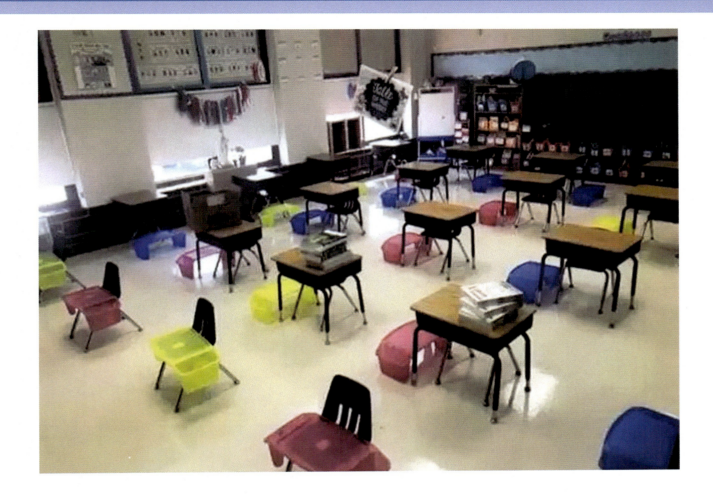

Physical Distancing Signs On The Street

Physical distancing sign is everywhere on the streets. This image portrays a sign on the sidewalk saying one person at a time. This demonstrates that we should respect the CDC guidelines. There is a reason for these signs to be everywhere that we can consider crowded.

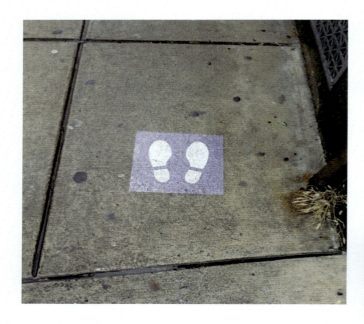

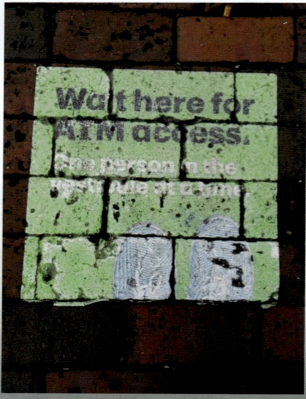

The Variants

Despite school openings, COVID-19 and its variants did not stop mutating. The variants are circulating inside classrooms and school halls, however, it is not yet a time to send students, teachers, and school staff home. Some school leaders are still waiting for orders In order to go home. **To be open or not to be open is never a question**. Meanwhile, COVID-19 Variants can be danced in the schools 'physical space. According to CDC here are some concerns encountered in my research: *"On July 27, 2021, CDC released updated guidance on the need for urgently increasing COVID-19 vaccination coverage and a recommendation for everyone in areas of substantial or high transmission to wear a mask in public indoor places, even if they are fully vaccinated. CDC issued this new guidance due to several concerning developments and newly emerging data signals."*

"In late June, the 7-day moving average of reported cases was around 12,000. On July 27, the 7-day moving average of cases reached over 60,000. This case rate looked more like the rate of cases we had seen before the vaccine was widely available."

".....new data began to emerge that the Delta variant was more infectious and was leading to increased transmissibility when compared with other variants, even in some vaccinated individuals".

> *"The Delta variant causes more infections and spreads faster than early forms of SARS-CoV-2, the virus that causes COVID-19.*

"The Delta variant is more contagious: The Delta variant is highly contagious, more than 2x as contagious as previous variants. **Some data suggest the Delta variant might cause more severe illness than previous variants in unvaccinated people**. In two different studies from Canada and Scotland, patients infected with the Delta variant were more likely to be hospitalized than patients infected with Alpha or the original virus that causes COVID-19. Even so, the vast majority of hospitalization and death caused by COVID-19 are in unvaccinated people."*

- "Unvaccinated people remain the greatest concern: *The greatest risk of transmission is among unvaccinated people who are much more likely to get infected, and therefore transmit the virus...People infected with the Delta variant, including fully vaccinated people with symptomatic breakthrough infections, can transmit the virus to others. CDC is continuing to assess data on whether fully vaccinated people with asymptomatic breakthrough infections can transmit the virus."*

"Fully vaccinated people with Delta variant breakthrough infections can spread the virus to others. However, vaccinated people appear to spread the virus for a shorter time: *For prior variants, lower amounts of viral genetic material were found in samples taken from fully vaccinated people who had breakthrough infections than from unvaccinated people with COVID-19. For people infected with the Delta variant, similar amounts viral genetic material has been found among both unvaccinated and fully vaccinated people. However, like prior variants, the amount of viral genetic material may go down faster in fully vaccinated people when compared to unvaccinated people. This means fully vaccinated people will likely spread the virus for less time than unvaccinated ...people."*

The vaccines nightmare!

- Many people are afraid of vaccines and they turn out to be against them. The reason for all of this nightmare thinking and beliefs are due to the fact that people sometimes hear a similar sentence on the news according to CDC, that: "... **But they are not 100% effective, and some fully vaccinated people will become infected (called a breakthrough infection) and experience illness.** *On the other hand, I quote this sentence from CDC:* "**Vaccines in the US are highly effective, including against the Delta variant.**"

"The COVID-19 vaccines approved or authorized in the United States are highly effective at preventing severe disease and death, including against the Delta variant. ..For all people, the vaccine provides the best protection against serious illness and death. Vaccines are playing a crucial role in limiting the spread of the virus and minimizing severe disease. Although vaccines are highly effective, but they are not perfect, and there will be vaccine breakthrough infections. Millions of Americans are vaccinated, and that number is growing. This means that even though the risk of breakthrough infections is low, there will be thousands of fully vaccinated people who become infected and able to infect others, especially with the surging spread of the Delta variant.

Vaccination is the best way to protect yourself, your family, and your community. High vaccination coverage will reduce the spread of the virus and help prevent new variants from emerging. CDC recommends that everyone aged 12 years and older get vaccinated as soon as possible."

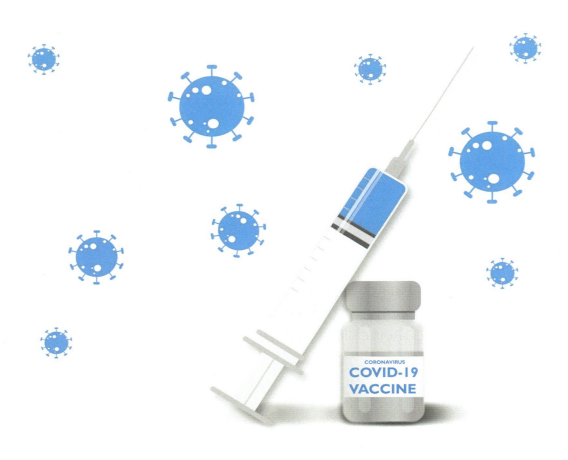

Omicron in Town!!!

Omicron is a variant that made us more alert. Some schools had to go back online.

The Omicron arrival in the USA

"CDC is working with state and local public health officials to monitor the spread of Omicron. As of December 20, 2021, Omicron has been detected in most states and territories and is rapidly increasing the proportion of COVID-19 cases it is causing"

As schools are keeping their doors open for students with mandates for rapid testing and or Vaccines, the Omicron variant is portrayed in the classrooms making and rising cases. Some Boston Public Schools are sending emails to parents in order to let them know about the new daily increased cases. This is what the CDC report about the Omicron variant: *"CDC has been collaborating with global public health and industry partners to learn about Omicron, as we continue to monitor its course. We don't yet know how easily it spreads, the severity of the illness causes, or how well available vaccines and medications work against it. The Omicron variant likely will spread more easily than the original SARS-CoV-2 virus and how easily Omicron spreads compared to Delta remains unknown. CDC expects that anyone with an Omicron infection can spread the virus to others, even if they are vaccinated or don't have symptoms.*

More data are needed to know if Omicron infections, and especially reinjection and Breakthrough, infections in people who are fully vaccinated, cause more severe illness or death than infection with other variants." Public Schools are sending letters to parents and caregivers every week, not to mention sometimes every day about rising cases in the schools and in addition to recommendations about how parents should proceed at home before sending their children to school.

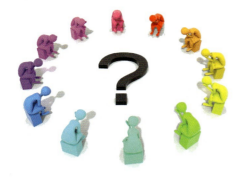

Why leave the schools open?

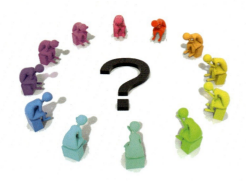

Home schooling appears to be tough.

Are the schools gaining anything by keeping the doors open and adding up the cases?

_____

_____

_____

_____

_____

_____

_____

_____

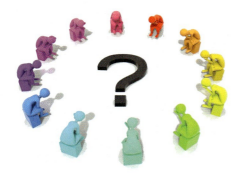

We have to experience and live with it!
For how long?

_____

_____

_____

_____

_____

_____

_____

_____

_____

Still in the nightmare of vaccines!

"Current vaccines are expected to protect against severe illness, hospitalizations, and death due to infection with the Omicron variant. However, breakthrough infections in people who are fully vaccinated are likely to occur. With other variants, like Delta, vaccines have remained effective at preventing severe illness, hospitalizations, and death. The recent emergence of Omicron further emphasizes the importance of vaccination and boosters."

Vaccines are crucial and they should be taken into consideration seriously. The virus is spreading rapidly as the variants continue to pop out continuously. This is a very serious aspect and the situation in the Education Realm and as well the world.

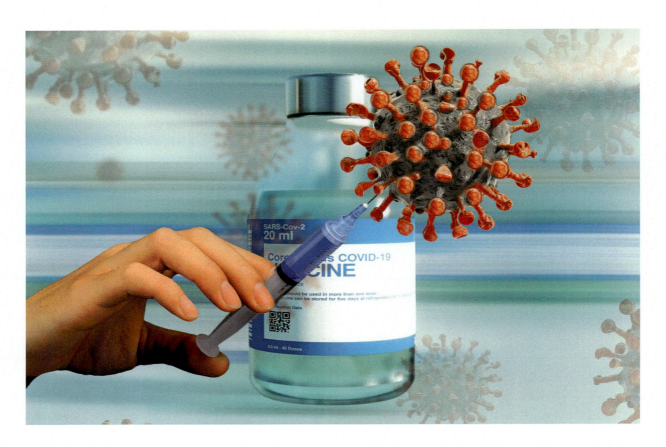

CDC highlights: "Scientists are currently investigating Omicron, including how protected fully vaccinated people will be against infection, hospitalization, and death. "DC recommends that everyone 5 years and older protect themselves from COVID-19 by getting fully vaccinated."

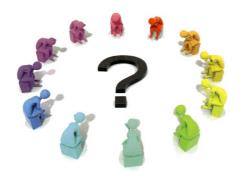 **What is your idea as parents about this?**

_____

_____

_____

_____

_____

_____

_____

_____

_____

_____

"CDC recommends that everyone ages 18 years and older should get a booster shot at least two months after their initial J&J/Janssen vaccine or six months after completing their primary COVID-19 vaccination series of Pfizer-BioNTech or Moderna."

"What CDC is Doing to Learn about Omicron?

CDC scientists are working with partners to gather data and virus samples that can be studied to answer important questions about the Omicron variant. Scientific experiments have already started. CDC will provide updates as soon as possible."

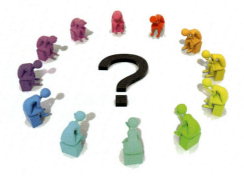

What updates could be possible updated?

_____

_____

_____

_____

_____

_____

_____

_____

_____

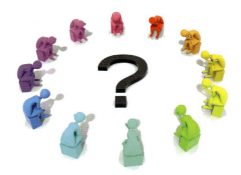

Is the world ready for more Variants?

_____

_____

_____

_____

_____

_____

_____

_____

_____

OBS:

Emergence of Omicron

> "**November 24, 2021**: A new variant of SARS-CoV-2, B.1.1.529, was reported to the World Health Organization (WHO). This new variant was first detected in specimens collected on November 11, 2021, in Botswana and on November 14, 2021, in South Africa. **November 26, 2021**: WHO named the B.1.1.529 Omicron and classified it as a Variant of Concern (VOC).November 30, 2021: The United States designated Omicron as a Variant of Concern. **December 1, 2021**: The first confirmed U.S. case of Omicron was identified."

The education realm turns out to be a world of changes and challenges. Schools all over the world had to take measures and be alert in terms of precautions and safety for the students and staff. Teachers had to work patiently and carefully with these measures in order to protect the students.

According to my research, I found that:

COVID-19 Prevention Strategies Most Important for Safe In-Person Learning in K-12 Schools is an important part of the infrastructure of communities. They provide safe and supportive learning environments for students that support social and emotional development, provide access to critical services, and improve life outcomes. They also employ people and enable parents, guardians, and caregivers to work. Though COVID-19 outbreaks have occurred in school settings, multiple studies have shown that transmission rates within school settings, when multiple prevention strategies are in place, are typically lower than— or similar to—community transmission levels. However, with the burden of COVID-19 transmission, protection against exposure remains essential in school settings."(https:// www.cdc.gov/coronavirus/2019-ncov/community/schools-childcare/k-12-guidance.html)

"Because of the highly transmissible nature of SARS-CoV-2, along with the mixing of vaccinated and unvaccinated people in schools, *CDC recommends universal indoor masking for all* students (ages 2 years and older), teachers, staff, and visitors to K-12 schools, regardless of vaccination status.*"

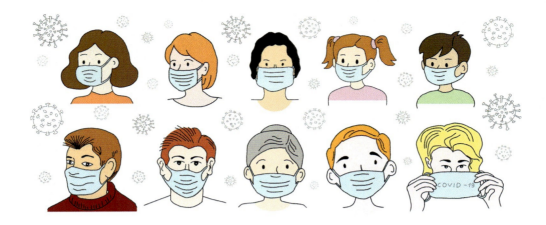

"Schools should work with local public health officials, consistent with applicable laws and regulations, including those related to privacy, to determine the additional prevention strategies needed in their area by monitoring levels of community transmission (low, moderate, substantial, or high) and local vaccine coverage, and use of screening testing to detect cases in K-12 schools. For example, with a low teacher, staff, or student vaccination rate, and without a screening testing program, schools might decide that they need to continue to maximize physical distancing or implement screening testing in addition to mask-wearing."

- "Schools should communicate their strategies and any changes in plans to teachers, staff, and families, and directly to older students, using accessible materials and communication channels, in a language and at a literacy level that teachers, staff, students and families understand *Prevention Strategies to Reduce Transmission of SARS-CoV-2 in Schools* *CDC recommends that all teachers, staff, and eligible students are vaccinated as soon as possible. However, schools have a mixed the population of both people who are fully vaccinated and people who are not fully vaccinated. This requires K-12 administrators to make decisions about the use of COVID-19 prevention strategies in their schools and is why CDC recommends universal indoor masking regardless of vaccination status at all levels of community transmission. Together with local public health officials, school administrators should consider multiple factors when they make decisions about implementing layered prevention strategies against COVID-19. Since schools typically serve their surrounding communities, decisions should be based on the school population, families, and students served, as well as their communities. The primary factors to consider include:*

Level of community transmission of COVID-19

COVID-19 vaccination coverage in the community and among students, teachers, and Staff Strain on health system capacity within the community.

"Accessibility of SARS-CoV-2 testing resources for students, teachers, and staff of a SARS-CoV-2 screening testing program for students, teachers, and staff. Testing provides an important layer of prevention, particularly in areas with substantial to high community transmission levels of COVID-19 outbreaks or increasing trends in the school or surrounding community."

"Ages of children served by K-12 schools and the associated social and behavioral factors that may affect the risk of transmission and the feasibility of different prevention strategies.(https://www.cdc.gov/coronavirus/2019-ncov/community/schools-childcare/k-12-guidance.html)"

Testing In Schools

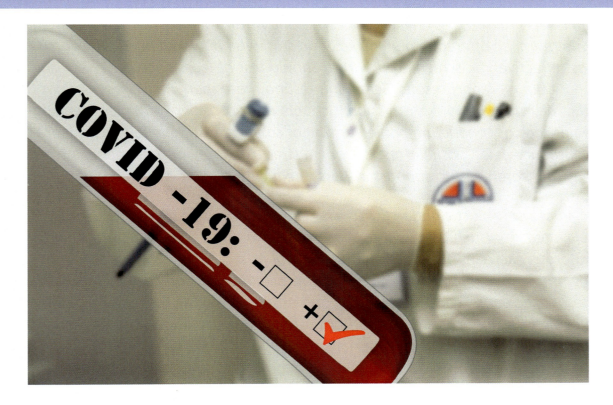

Updated Jan. 6, 2022

Screening Testing

Testing in school has been one of the method that can help us Educator feel safe in terms of having classes among students coming from different houses.

According to my, research CDC highlights that: *"Screening testing identifies infected people, including those with or without symptoms (or before the development of symptoms) who may be contagious, so that measures can be taken to prevent further transmission. In K-12 schools, screening testing can help promptly identify and isolate cases, initiate quarantine and identify clusters to help reduce the risk to in-person education. Decisions regarding screening testing may be made at the state or local level. A screening test may be most valuable in areas with substantial or high community transmission levels, in areas with low vaccination coverage, and in schools where other prevention strategies are not implemented. More frequent testing can increase effectiveness, but the feasibility of increased testing in schools needs to be considered. Screening testing should be done in a way that ensures the ability to maintain the confidentiality of results and protect student, teacher, and staff privacy. ..."*

"Screening testing can be used to help evaluate and adjust prevention strategies and provide added protection for schools that are not able to provide optimal physical distance between students. At a minimum, screening testing should be offered to students who have not been fully vaccinated when community transmission is at moderate, substantial, or high levels (Table 1). At any level of community transmission, screening testing should, at a minimum, be offered to all teachers and staff who have not been fully vaccinated. To be most effective, the screening program should test at least once per week, and rapidly (within 24 hours) report results. Screening testing more than once a week might be more effective at interrupting transmission. Schools may consider multiple screening testing strategies such as conducting pooled testing of cohorts. Testing in low-prevalence settings might produce false positive results, but testing can provide an important prevention strategy and safety net to support in-person education."

"To facilitate safe participation in sports, extracurricular activities, and other activities with elevated risk (such as activities that involve singing or shouting, band participation, and vigorous exercise that could lead to forceful or increased exhalation), schools should consider implementing screening testing for participants. Schools can routinely test student-athletes, participants, coaches, trainers, and other people (such as adult volunteers) who could come into close contact with others during these activities. Schools should consider implementing screening testing of participants up to 24 hours before sporting, competition, or extracurricular events. Schools can use different screening testing strategies for lower-risk sports. High-risk sports and extracurricular activities should be virtual or canceled in areas of high community transmission unless all participants are fully vaccinated."(https:// www.cdc.gov/coronavirus/2019-ncov/community/schools-childcare/k-12-guidance.html)

Table 1. Screening Testing Recommendations for K-12 Schools by Level of Community Transmission

	Low Transmission[1] Blue	Moderate Transmission Yellow	Substantial Transmission Orange	High Transmission Red
Students	Do not need to screen students.	**Offer screening testing for students**[4] at least once per week.		
Teachers and staff	**Offer screening testing for teachers and staff**[4] at least once per week.			
High risk sports and activities	**Recommend screening testing for high-risk sports**[2] **and extracurricular activities**[3] at least once per week.		**Recommend screening testing for high-risk sports and extracurricular activities** twice per week.	**Cancel or hold high-risk sports and extracurricular activities virtually** to protect in-person learning.
Low- and intermediate-risk sports	Do not need to screen students participating in low- and intermediate-risk sports.[2]	**Recommend screening testing for low- and intermediate-risk sports** at least once per week.		

We all are aware now staying Home while sick is best for us and others, we need to take this recommendation from CDC seriously. Below is what CDC recommends:

"Staying Home When Sick and Getting Tested

Students, teachers, and staff who have symptoms of infectious illness, such as influenza (flu) or COVID-19, should stay home and be referred to their healthcare provider for testing and care, regardless of vaccination status. Staying home when sick with COVID-19 is essential to keep COVID-19 infections out of schools and prevent their spread to others."

"In the K-12 school setting, CDC recommends ending isolation based on timing after symptom onset or positive test result (if asymptomatic). Everyone with COVID-19 should stay home and isolated away from other people for at least 5 full days (day 0 is the first day of symptoms or the day of the positive viral test for asymptomatic persons). They should wear a well-fitting mask when around others at home and in public for an additional 5 days. People who have symptoms can end isolation after 5 full days only if they are fever-free for 24 hours without the use of fever-reducing medication and if other symptoms have improved. They should continue to wear a well-fitting mask around others at home and in public for 5 additional days".

"Schools should also allow flexible, non-punitive, and supportive paid sick leave policies and practices that encourage sick workers to stay home without fear of retaliation, loss of pay, or loss of employment level and provide excused absences for students who are sick. Employers should ensure that workers are aware of and understand these policies. . If a school does not have a routine screening testing program, the ability to do rapid testing on-site could facilitate COVID-19 diagnosis and inform the need for quarantine of close contacts and isolation."

"Schools should educate teachers, staff, and families about when they and their children should stay home and when they can return to school. During the COVID-19 pandemic, it is essential that parents keep children home if they are showing signs and symptoms of COVID-19 and get them promptly tested, and notify the school if they test positive. Getting tested for COVID-19 when symptoms are compatible with COVID-19 will help with rapid contact tracing and prevent the possible spread at schools, especially if key prevention strategies (masking and distancing) are not in use". https://www.cdc.gov/coronavirus/2019-ncov/community/schools-childcare/k-12-guidance.html#mask-use

Students and staff were asked to be tested in schools even though they presented no symptoms. Vaccinations were also required and mandatory by CDC in order to turn the school environment safe. As it is said below:

"As schools go back to in-person learning, some may offer regular COVID-19 testing for students and staff. This means testing is offered regularly, even for people who do not have symptoms of COVID-19. Many schools will also offer to test for people with symptoms of COVID-19 or who have been exposed to someone with COVID-19. Schools do not need to require a negative test result for students, teachers, and staff to return to school after breaks. Students, teachers, and staff who travel during breaks should follow CDC testing recommendations for domestic and international travel.(https:// www.CDC.gov/coronavirus/2019-testing/symptoms.)

"Regular testing, in addition to COVID-19 vaccination, is a safe, effective way to help prevent the spread of COVID-19 and help keep schools open for in-person learning. Many people with COVID-19, especially children and teens, don't have symptoms but can still spread the virus, so regular testing helps find people who have the virus before it can spread to others. This is especially important for children who are not yet vaccinated against COVID-19, families and staff with younger children at home, those at risk for getting seriously sick from COVID-19, and those who are not fully vaccinated against COVID-19. Finding who has the virus early means steps can be taken to prevent COVID-19 from spreading and causing an outbreak, so schools can stay open. Regular testing also means parents or guardians get notified if their child tests positive, allowing them to plan for treatment and take steps to protect the rest of the family from COVID-19.(https://www.CDC.gov/coronavirus/2019-testing/symptoms)."

"The tests are free, quick, and easy and will help to tell if students or staff have COVID-19, even if they do not have symptoms. Schools may choose to use either a nasal test, using a swab for the lower part of the inner nostril, or a saliva test, which takes a saliva (spit) sample. The nasal test is not painful and does **not** use the longer swab that reaches higher into the nose. Staff will not be tested without consent. Students will not be tested without the consent of both the student and their guardian..(https://www. CDC.gov/coronavirus/2019-testing/symptoms)".

COVID-19 Symptoms

People with COVID-19 have had a wide range of symptoms reported – ranging from mild symptoms to severe illness. Symptoms may appear 2-14 days after exposure to the virus. Anyone can have mild to severe symptoms. People with these symptoms may have COVID-19: (https://www.CDC.gov/coronavirus/2019-testing/symptoms)"

- Fever or chills

- Cough

- Shortness of breath or difficulty breathing

- Fatigue

- Muscle or body aches

- Headache

- New loss of taste or smell

- Sore throat

- Congestion or runny nose

- Nausea or vomiting

- Diarrhea

NEA beliefs that all schools, especially in communities with substantial or high rates of COVID-19, should have in place screening testing to help stop the spread of COVID-19.

In fact, students, teachers, parents and school staff would feel more secure by knowing that they are being tested and free to go for the day. Teachers should be aware of testing and make sure all students are being tested before class for this period of time things may change to the point that Educators could be told that testing or wearing masks are not mandatory anymore we will wait for the changes and we will be changing according to what we are told.

"Screening COVID-19 testing, sometimes called asymptomatic testing, involves testing everyone, or more likely, a randomly selected sample of individuals in a group. Screening testing is intended to identify infections in people with no known exposure who are asymptomatic or have not yet developed symptoms. NEA recognizes that screening

testing programs in schools can be complex, including requiring adjustments to school routines, work duties, and schedules." (htt://www.whitehouse.gov/briefing-room/ statements-releases/2022/01/12).

"CDC also recognizes the role test-to-stay strategies an approach to testing that combines contact tracing and repeated testing of asymptomatic people--can play in keeping students who have been exposed to COVID-19 in school instead of quarantine. For more information, see the section below on steps to reduce the burden of quarantine. *To double the capacity of testing available in schools, provide more guidance on "test-to-stay"*

Omicron Alert!

As a professor and writer, I found myself very interested in the new upcoming news about Omicron in order to be updated with Omicron waves so that I can inform my students. According to NEA media-center press-/release/blank, these are some information that I collected:

"WASHINGTON — This morning the Biden administration announced new nationwide to mitigate the spread of Omicron".

"The following statement can be attributed to NEA President Becky Pringle: "We applaud the Biden administration for heeding the call of educators across the nation to center our school communities in the pandemic response strategy and providing even more resources to keep our students, educators, and all their families safe. The National Education Association is already mobilizing its members and leaders to work with schools as well as state and local governments to take advantage of the new testing resources".

"Omicron has brought a wave of cases to our school communities, and this increase in testing capacity will go a long way in slowing the spread and keeping our students and educators are healthy. However, it is still paramount that states use available American Rescue Plan funds for all the safety measures we know work, the personnel needed to implement them, and for paid leave when staff is required to isolate and quarantine. We must continue to focus on a layered the strategy of vaccinations and boosters, masks, proper ventilation, and testing policies to save lives and help ensure the well-being of students and educators as they continue to safely learn and work in person together."

The National Education Association is the nation's largest professional employee organization, representing more than 3 million elementary and secondary teachers, higher education faculty, education support professionals, school administrators, retired educators, students preparing to become teachers, healthcare workers, and public employees.(https://www.nea.org/about-nea/media-center/press-releases/blank).

"To wear a mask or not to wear". It should be never a question.

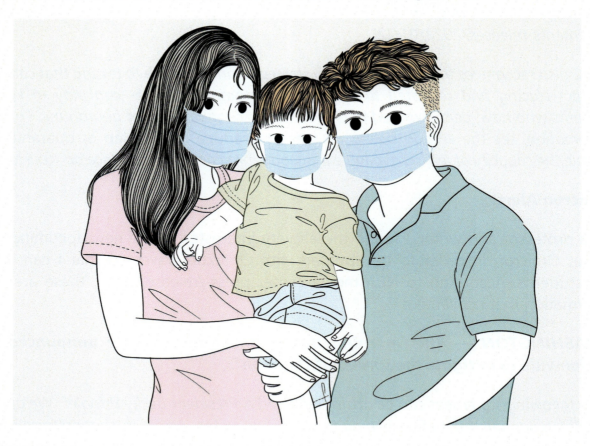

What do you think?

_____

_____

_____

_____

_____

_____

_____

_____

_____

References

- ls://www.nea.org/about-nea/media-center/press-releases/blank)

- (htt://www.whitehouse.gov/briefing-room/statements releases/2022/01/12)https://coronavirusexplained.ukri.org/en/article/pub0006

- U.S. Department of Health & Human Services

- USA.govCDC Website Exit Disclaimer external

- http://www.euro.who.int /en/healthtopics/health-emergencies/coronavirus-COVID

- https://www.cdc.gov/coronavirus/2019ncov/variants/deltavariant.
html?s_cid=11504:delta%20variant%20covid%20vaccine%20efficacy:sem.
ga:p:RG:GM:gen:PTN:FY21

- **NEA comment on Tik Tok challenge threatening violence at schools:** *Pringle: "These types of threats and social media trends are very disturbing and in no way amusing"* **:By: Staci Maiers: Published: 12/16/2021 Last Updated: 12/16/2021**

Celeste Busser: Published: 01/12/2022

Let's find out more on the next Invisible Magazine.

MORE UPDATES NEXT CHRISTMAS 2022

Printed in the United States
by Baker & Taylor Publisher Services